ESSENTIAL GUIDE TO SEBORRHEIC DERMATITIS

Understanding, Managing, and Thriving:
An In-Depth Exploration of Seborrheic Dermatitis

DR. CASEY LOREN

DISCLAIMER

This book's content is only meant to be used for general informative purposes. Although the author has taken great care to ensure the content is accurate and thorough, no warranties or assurances on the information's accuracy, correctness, or reliability are provided. It is recommended that readers employ their own judgment and discretion when applying any material found in this book to their particular situation.

The information in this book is not intended to replace professional advice, nor is the author an expert in any of the subjects covered. It is recommended that readers consult with experienced professionals regarding any particular issues or concerns.

Any name that may be mentioned or referred in this book does not imply endorsement, recommendation, or relationship on the part of the author with any person, entity, good, website, or association. These references are made only for informational purposes and are not meant to be taken as recommendations or endorsements.

The information contained in this book may cause readers to suffer loss or damage, for which the author disclaims all obligation and accountability. The only people accountable for the decisions and actions taken by readers using the information presented are themselves.

Any names, characters, companies, locations, activities, occasions, and incidents referenced in this book are either made up or the result of the author's imagination. Any likeness to real people, living or dead, or to real things is entirely coincidental.

This book's content may change at any time, without prior notice, according to the author. The onus is on the reader to verify whether there have been any updates or revisions.

The reader accepts the conditions of this disclaimer by reading this book. Please do not read this book or use its contents if you do not agree to these terms.   5

Table of Contents

CHAPTER 1

SEBORRHOEIC DERMATITIS: A COMPREHENSIVE OVERVIEW

Introduction and Definition

Red, itchy, flaky patches are the hallmarks of seborrhoeic dermatitis, a prevalent skin condition that usually strikes regions abundant in sebaceous glands, such as the scalp, face, and upper chest. Scaly spots on the face, especially around the nose, ears, and eyebrows, or dandruff on the scalp are common symptoms.

Reasons and Initiators

Genetics, hormonal shifts, stress, and specific skin microbes (such as Malassezia yeast) are thought to have a role in the development of seborrhoeic dermatitis, however, the actual reason is still unknown. Some medical diseases, such as Parkinson's disease or HIV/AIDS, as well as changes in the weather, greasy skin, and strong soaps and detergents can all act as triggers.

Typical Signs

Seborrhoeic dermatitis manifests itself on the skin as redness, itching, peeling, and the development of crusty or oily scales. There is a wide range in the intensity and recurrence of these symptoms.

Methods for Diagnosis

A physical examination of the skin affected and a review of the patient's medical history are the usual tools used by doctors to diagnose seborrhoeic dermatitis. To rule out other possible conditions, additional testing, such as a skin biopsy, may be necessary in certain instances.

Setting It Apart from Alternative Skin Disorders

Seborrhoeic dermatitis differs from eczema and psoriasis, two other skin disorders, in terms of its unique symptoms, site of manifestation, and microscopic appearance.

Effects on Living Standards

Even while seborrhoeic dermatitis isn't life-threatening, it can be embarrassing and debilitating if it's extensive or has persisted for a long time.

Trends and Characteristics

Anyone can get seborrhoeic dermatitis; however, adults, those with oily skin, and those with specific medical disorders are more likely to experience it.

Looking back at the past

Ancient medical writings describe skin disorders that are similar to seborrhoeic dermatitis, which has a history that goes back centuries. Our knowledge and ability to treat this problem have both been enhanced by the development of new medical technologies.

New Findings and Progress in the Field

Researchers are constantly trying to figure out what causes seborrhoeic dermatitis, how to treat it better, and whether there are any connections to other health issues.

Expectations and Trends for the Future

Possible developments in the care of seborrhoeic dermatitis in the future include more effective patient education and support services, topical medication advancements, and individualized treatment plans based on hereditary characteristics.

CHAPTER 2

SEBORRHOEIC DERMATITIS: A VISIBLE EXAM

The ABCs of Skin Structure:

Seborrhoeic dermatitis can be better understood with a basic familiarity with skin anatomy. These three layers—the epidermis, dermis, and hypodermis—make up the skin. The epidermis is the most common site of seborrhoeic dermatitis, which affects regions abundant in sebaceous glands. Oily sebum is produced by these glands and lubricates the hair and skin.

Function of the Sebaceous Gland:

An important part of seborrhoeic dermatitis is sebaceous glands. They help maintain the skin's protective barrier by producing sebum, which is rich in lipids and fatty acids. Nevertheless, seborrhoeic dermatitis can arise when sebum is either overproduced or has an abnormal nature.

The Workings of the Hair Follicle:

Seborrhoeic dermatitis involves the hair follicles as they are associated with sebaceous glands. When there is an imbalance, the yeast Malassezia, which is typically found in hair follicles, can worsen the problem.

What the Immune System Does:

In seborrhoeic dermatitis, the immune system is very important. Inflammation and the growth of

Malassezia, which cause redness, itching, and flaking, might be triggered by an aberrant immune response.

The Impact of the Microbiome:

Seborrhoeic dermatitis is impacted by the skin's microbiome, which comprises various microorganisms such as bacteria and fungi. The skin's protective mechanisms can be affected by changes in the microbiome, which can lead to the development of the disorder.

The Role of Heredity:

There may be a hereditary component to seborrhoeic dermatitis. An increased risk of developing the condition may be associated with certain genetic variations that influence the immune response, sebum production, or the skin's capacity to sustain a balanced microbiome.

The Role of Hormones:

Mood swings like those that happen during pregnancy, puberty, or hormone imbalances might impact seborrhoeic dermatitis. The skin's reaction to Malassezia, immunological function, and sebum production can all be influenced by hormones.

Potential Environmental Factors:

Environmental variables such as fluctuating humidity, temperature swings, pollution, and contact with certain allergens or chemicals can either cause or worsen seborrhoeic dermatitis. One or more of these things might encourage the growth of microbes or damage the skin's protective barrier.

Relationships with the Mind:

Seborrhoeic dermatitis can be impacted by psychological variables such as stress, worry, and depression. Symptoms may become more severe as a result of stress hormones' effects on immunological function and inflammation.

A Comprehensive View of Dermatitis:

Diet, lifestyle, stress management, and skincare habits are all part of a comprehensive approach to seborrhoeic dermatitis. Complementing traditional treatments with complementary therapies like mindfulness techniques, probiotics, and herbal remedies may help maintain healthy skin.

Healthcare providers can improve outcomes for patients with seborrhoeic dermatitis by gaining a thorough grasp of these factors and using that knowledge to create individualized plans for treatment and maintenance.

CHAPTER 3

SIGNS AND SYMPTOMS IN THE CLINIC

Eczema of the Scalp:

Common symptoms of seborrhoeic dermatitis include redness, itching, and flaking of the scalp, which is also known as scalp dermatitis. Scalp irritation ranging from moderate dandruff to severe can occur. Itching and tenderness are common complaints from patients, and they may even scratch in an attempt to alleviate the pain.

Head and Face Eczema:

The most common locations affected by red, oily patches with fine scales in seborrhoeic dermatitis of the face are the eyebrows, the sides of the nose, and the space between the upper lip and the nose (nasolabial folds). It can also spread to men's beards, foreheads, and cheeks. Some people may have feelings of shame or self-consciousness due to the condition's obviousness.

Eye and Ear Involvement:

Redness, scaling, and itching can be seen in areas affected by seborrhoeic dermatitis, such as the ears and eyelids. In other areas, like the ear canal and the lashes of the eyes, the scales could be oily and yellowish. To prevent further irritation and problems, it is important to manage seborrhoeic dermatitis away from the eyes.

Wounds on the trunk and legs:

Although it is more frequent on the scalp and face, seborrhoeic dermatitis can also appear on the trunk and limbs. Red, scaly patches or more widespread redness and inflammation are two ways lesions on the limbs and trunk might manifest. Particularly in places where the skin folds or rubs against garments, patients may feel itching and pain.

Diaper Rash Caused by Seborrhea:

Babies and toddlers can develop seborrhoeic dermatitis in a variety of forms, one of which is nappy dermatitis. In the diaper region, it shows up as redness, scaling, and occasionally teary sores. Careful assessment by a healthcare professional is crucial for correct diagnosis and treatment because this condition can be hard to distinguish from other types of nappy dermatitis.

Revamp Your Nails:

Changes such as ridges, discoloration, and thickening can occur in the nails due to seborrhoeic dermatitis, which is less prevalent. When assessing patients with anomalies in their nails, healthcare personnel should keep in mind that seborrhoeic dermatitis can sometimes include the nails, even though this is not always the case.

Secondary infections and other complications:

Secondary fungal or bacterial infections are a possible consequence of seborrhoeic dermatitis. The skin's protective barrier can be compromised by scratching, making it easier for germs to invade the skin. Reddening, swelling, discomfort, and discharge are some of the symptoms that may accompany these illnesses. The best way to stop secondary infections from getting worse is to treat them right away.

Nonstandard Displays:

Symptoms of seborrhoeic dermatitis can be similar to those of eczema or psoriasis, two common skin disorders. More extensive engagement, non-standard distribution patterns, or the absence of traditional scales are all examples of atypical presentations. Healthcare personnel need to be on the lookout for seborrhoeic dermatitis, particularly in situations that are difficult or unclear.

Distinctions in Humans of All Ages:

Age can have a role in how seborrhoeic dermatitis manifests. The diaper region and the scalp (cradle cap) are common sites of infection in newborns. Aside from the scalp, the face, trunk, and limbs can also be involved in children. While the illness can impact other locations, it most typically affects adults' scalps and faces. To diagnose and treat patients effectively, it is helpful to understand these age-related differences.

Obstacles and Factors to Consider in Diagnostics:

Seborrhoeic dermatitis can be difficult to diagnose, particularly in cases when it shows no symptoms at all or when it coexists with other skin issues. To develop a definitive diagnosis, doctors must take into account the patient's medical history, and current symptoms, and, in some cases, conduct supplementary tests such as skin biopsies or cultures. Psoriasis, eczema, tinea infections, and other possible illnesses necessitate a comprehensive evaluation to determine the best course of treatment.

CHAPTER 4

THE SIGNIFICANCE OF MEDICAL HISTORY

The diagnosis and evaluation of seborrhoeic dermatitis depend on a thorough medical history. This aids in the detection of risk factors, such as a history of skin disorders in the family, previous illnesses (particularly those affecting the immune system), and medications (particularly those containing corticosteroids or immunosuppressants). To understand how a disease develops and how therapy works, it is crucial to get a thorough history of symptoms, including how long they lasted, what triggered them, and how the patient responded to earlier treatments.

Important Points of a Physical Examination

A comprehensive physical examination is crucial for evaluating seborrheic dermatitis. Important considerations include evaluating the extent and location of lesions, as well as checking often affected areas such as the ears, chest, intertriginous regions, and scalp (particularly nasolabial folds and eyebrows). Seborrhoeic dermatitis is characterized by redness, scaling, and oily areas; also, you should check for secondary infections and other skin issues that can be present.

Imaging and Dermoscopy Methods

Seborrhoeic dermatitis can be better diagnosed by dermoscopy, which shows vascular patterns, follicular plugs, and yellowish scales. To help with differential diagnosis and treatment planning, imaging techniques such as reflectance confocal microscopy can give precise views of dermal and epidermal components.

Examinations in a Scientific Setting

Although skin biopsies and fungal cultures are the mainstays of clinical diagnosis for seborrhoeic dermatitis, they may be necessary in situations that do not respond to treatment or when other possible diagnoses are being considered. These tests are useful for ruling out overlapping dermatoses, fungal infections, and psoriasis.

Approach to Diagnosis

To narrow down the possible causes of seborrhoeic dermatitis, doctors look for symptoms that are similar to those of psoriasis, atopic dermatitis, tinea infections, or rosacea. The degree of pruritus, the location of lesions, the presence or absence of greasy scales, and the efficacy of treatments are important indicators of differentiation.

Scales for Assessing Severity

The Seborrhoeic Dermatitis Area and Severity Index (SDASI) is one such severity grading system that aids in the standardization of illness assessment and the monitoring of therapy response. To determine the severity of the condition and the best course of treatment, they look at indicators including erythema, scaling, and the total area of the affected body.

Self-Evaluation Instruments for Patients

The Dermatology Life Quality Index (DLQI) and other patient self-assessment instruments allow patients to monitor their symptoms, reactions to treatment, and the overall effect on their daily lives. Care that is patient-centered and treatment adherence are both helped by these technologies.

Psychosocial Effects Evaluation

Seborrhoeic dermatitis can have a major influence on quality of life, self-esteem, and social relationships; thus, it is crucial to evaluate the psychosocial impact. Those suffering from serious mental illness or emotional pain may benefit from psychological evaluations and therapy.

Partnerships between medical experts (such as dermatologists and allergists)

To effectively manage seborrhoeic dermatitis, it is crucial to work with other medical specialists such as dermatologists and allergists. While allergists may help find and treat the sources of an allergic reaction, dermatologists are experts in making diagnoses and providing long-term care.

Strategies for Patient Education

The management of seborrhoeic dermatitis relies heavily on patient education. The chronic nature of the problem, potential triggers (such as stress, harsh soaps, and cold weather), correct skincare regimens, medication adherence, and medical attention for worsening symptoms or consequences should be part of the patient education strategy.

Clinicians can improve outcomes for patients with seborrhoeic dermatitis by incorporating these elements into their practice, which aids in diagnosis, evaluation, and management.

CHAPTER 5

METHODS FOR TREATMENT

Aesthetic Treatments

To control seborrhoeic dermatitis, topical treatments are essential. Direct topical applications of medicinal shampoos, creams, and lotions are among these. Medications that reduce inflammation or antifungal agents are common active components in these products.

Fungal Antifungal Drugs

Seborrhoeic dermatitis is treated with antifungal medicines because it is a fungal infection. Selenium sulfide, ciclopirox, and ketoconazole are common antifungal medications. The Malassezia yeast, which is commonly linked to the illness, can be inhibited by these drugs.

Medication for Reducing Inflammation

Seborrhoeic dermatitis symptoms such as redness, swelling, and itching can be alleviated with the use of anti-inflammatory drugs. Topical versions of corticosteroids are frequently used for inflammation control. Because of the potential for adverse consequences with long-term usage, powerful steroids are typically used only when necessary or in conjunction with other treatments.

Inhibitors of Calcineurin

Tacrolimus and tacrolimus are examples of calcineurin inhibitors that are used to treat seborrhoeic dermatitis. The anti-inflammatory and immune-modulating effects of these drugs are what make them effective. When corticosteroids aren't a good long-term option, they're utilized.

Pills for the Mouth

If the condition is severe or if topical treatments are not working, the patient may be given medication orally. To combat Malassezia yeast systemically, you can use oral antifungal medications such as fluconazole or itraconazole. To manage severe inflammation, oral corticosteroids may also be recommended for shorter durations.

Treatments Involving Light and Phototherapy

When other therapies for seborrhoeic dermatitis have failed, phototherapy, which includes both broad-spectrum UVB light and narrowband UVB light, can be helpful. Inflammation and the rate of skin cell proliferation can be reduced by light-based treatments.

Alternative and Complementary Medicine

The management of seborrhoeic dermatitis may lead some people to investigate complementary and alternative medicine. Herbal treatments, essential oils, and nutritional supplements may fall within this category. Although these methods have helped some people, it is important to talk to a doctor before using them on yourself because their effectiveness and safety might vary greatly.

Changes to One's Way of Life

To alleviate seborrhoeic dermatitis, one might make some changes to their way of life. Some examples of this include eating well, not overstressing oneself, using mild skin care products, and avoiding harsh chemicals and soaps. Because stress can worsen skin disorders, it can be especially important to manage stress levels.

Food and Drink Factors

Seborrhoeic dermatitis is not caused by any one meal, but a healthy diet can help keep your skin in good condition. Some people have flare-ups in response to particular meals or eating habits; keeping a food diary might help pinpoint these triggers.

Approaches to Management for the Future

Individualized treatment plans often include a mix of medicines for the long-term management of seborrhoeic dermatitis. Methods such as making lifestyle changes, using medicated shampoos or creams on an as-needed basis, and scheduling frequent appointments with a dermatologist to assess response and make any necessary adjustments to treatment may be part of this regimen.

CHAPTER 6

DETAILS TO KEEP IN MIND WHEN DEALING WITH SEBORRHOEIC DERMATITIS

Cases in Children:

The symptoms and signs of seborrhoeic dermatitis in kids can vary from those in adults. While it most frequently impacts the scalp ("cradle cap"), it has the potential to spread to the neck, face, and diaper region as well. Babies' sensitive skin requires mild, doctor-approved treatments. One way to alleviate discomfort is to use gentle, fragrance-free treatments and keep the afflicted areas clean. It is critical to have regular checkups with a doctor to make sure you are getting the right treatment and to rule out any potential problems.

Lessened skin barrier function, co-morbidities, and drug interactions make seborrhoeic dermatitis more difficult to treat in the elderly. It is critical to pick anti-aging remedies with care. If you check your skin often, you can detect problems sooner, which means you can get treatment faster and have a better quality of life.

Pregnancy and Hormonal fluctuations:

Hormonal fluctuations during pregnancy might cause seborrhoeic dermatitis to fluctuate. While some women may find an improvement in their symptoms, others may find that they get worse. When making treatment decisions during pregnancy, it is crucial to consult with a healthcare professional to ensure the safety of both the mother and the unborn child. The problem might be further complicated by hormonal changes after giving birth, which necessitates constant attention.

People with impaired immune systems, such as those living with HIV/AIDS or on immunosuppressive medication, are at a higher risk of developing severe and long-lasting seborrhoeic dermatitis. For thorough care and best results, dermatologists and other healthcare professionals must work closely together, and treatment methods may need to be more aggressive.

The psychological effects of seborrhoeic dermatitis, include the potential to lower self-esteem and diminish quality of life, necessitating the development of coping mechanisms. Some ways to deal with health issues include learning more about the disease, developing skills to deal with stress, and connecting with others who understand what you're going through. Part of providing comprehensive care is helping patients cope emotionally with their chronic skin condition.

Complex management issues arise when seborrhoeic dermatitis occurs alongside other skin disorders such as psoriasis or rosacea. To effectively control symptoms and enhance outcomes, individualized treatment strategies that take all conditions into account at the same time are crucial. Thorough care is guaranteed by consistent follow-ups and open lines of communication among professionals.

Seborrhoeic dermatitis can be worsened by working in certain jobs or in surroundings where there is a high concentration of allergens, irritants, or humidity. Occupational health assessments can help reduce the impact on persons working in these situations by recommending skin protection measures and suitable skincare regimens. Another way to create a welcoming workplace is to raise awareness about the illness between coworkers and employers.

Climate change, increased humidity, and pollution are just a few examples of environmental and travel-related variables that might aggravate seborrhoeic dermatitis. It is possible to alleviate travel-related symptoms by taking preventative actions, such as bringing appropriate skincare products, sticking to a regular skincare routine, and staying away from recognized triggers. For tailored recommendations based on specific requirements, it's recommended to consult a dermatologist before to trip.

Participating in sports or other physically demanding activities, particularly those that involve perspiration and friction, can cause or aggravate seborrhoeic dermatitis. You can lessen the likelihood of breakouts by following a pre-workout skincare regimen, wearing clothes that absorb perspiration, and quickly washing off and drying off after exercise. It is also vital to avoid irritants and clogged pores by using skincare products that are not comedogenic.

As a visible skin ailment, seborrhoeic dermatitis carries with it the social stigma that can affect one's self-esteem and relationships with others. Healthcare providers loved ones, and friends can all play an important role in providing both emotional and practical support as you work to manage your disease. One way to combat the shame and ignorance around seborrhoeic dermatitis is to raise awareness about the condition.

CHAPTER 7

INNOVATING AND USING TECHNOLOGY: A CRITICAL ROLE

Electronic Health Records and Online Consultations:

By facilitating distant discussions between patients and medical professionals, telemedicine has transformed healthcare, particularly dermatology. People suffering from seborrhoeic dermatitis can now get professional guidance and treatment without having to physically visit a clinic. Those in more rural locations, in particular, benefit from virtual consultations because of the increased accessibility, decreased waiting times, and overall convenience they provide.

Portable Self-Monitoring Apps:

The symptoms of seborrhoeic dermatitis can be better managed with the help of mobile apps that record flare-ups, medication compliance, and skincare practices. Better outcomes and more effective communication between patients and healthcare providers are the results of their enabling patients to take an active role in managing their disease.

Dermatology and Wearable Technology:

Seborrhoeic dermatitis-related physiological factors, including skin moisture levels and temperature variations, can be tracked via wearable devices like skin sensors. Early diagnosis of exacerbations and personalized treatment strategies are both made possible with this data.

The Role of AI and ML in the Diagnosis Process:

Machine learning algorithms and artificial intelligence (AI) sift through massive databases of dermatological pictures and patient data to aid in the diagnosis of seborrhoeic dermatitis. Improved diagnostic accuracy, faster evaluations, and decision-making support are all benefits of these technological advancements for the healthcare industry.

Findings from Big Data:

The epidemiology, treatment results, and patient profiles of seborrhoeic dermatitis can be better understood with the use of big data analytics, which extract useful information from massive datasets. Continuous improvement in care delivery is driven by these insights, which inform evidence-based approaches.

Exploring New Drugs and Conducting Clinical Trials:

New drug formulations and tailored therapy are changing the game when treating seborrhoeic dermatitis. Novel therapeutic approaches are made possible by the evaluation of the safety and effectiveness of novel drugs in clinical trials.

Potential Uses of Nanotechnology:

Targeted medication delivery systems and skin barrier strengthening are two potential dermatological uses of nanotechnology. To maximize therapy efficacy and minimize negative effects, nano-sized particles can penetrate epidermal layers effectively.

Methods for Customised Medical Care:

Genetic factors, microbiome composition, and lifestyle habits are just a few of the particular patient features that personalized medicine takes into account when developing treatment strategies. This method reduces side effects while increasing treatment efficacy.

Important Moral Factors:

Patient confidentiality, data protection, fair technology access, and informed permission for innovative treatments are all important ethical factors to consider when managing seborrhoeic dermatitis. To protect patients' rights and well-being, healthcare practitioners must negotiate these complex ethical landscapes.

Looking Ahead: Potential Paths

With continuous improvements in technology, research, and patient-centered approaches, the future of seborrhoeic dermatitis therapy is bright. Integrated digital platforms for complete dermatological care, precision medicines, and AI-driven predictive models are all possible future advances. To make these potentials a reality and improve outcomes for people with seborrhoeic dermatitis, stakeholders must continue to collaborate.

CHAPTER 8

EYEWITNESS ACCOUNTS AND PATIENT FEEDBACK

Tales of Survival and Resilience:

Experiences, obstacles, and victories create each person's journey with seborrhoeic dermatitis in their special way. The illness may have been present in some people's lives from a young age, while it may have taken longer to diagnose others. No matter when it started, telling one's story of coping and recovering can help others going through the same things. Narratives like these typically focus on the ups and downs of dealing with seborrhoeic dermatitis, from the first shock and frustration to the final acceptance and adaption. Their ability to overcome adversity and discover solutions that work to alleviate symptoms and enhance quality of life is truly inspiring.

Problems That People Deal With Every Day:

Seborrhoeic dermatitis is a chronic skin condition that can greatly affect a person's quality of life. Individuals afflicted with this ailment may encounter challenges that necessitate continuous treatment and adaptation; these may range from the physical discomfort of itching, redness, and peeling skin to the mental burden of coping with visible symptoms. Managing one's self-esteem and confidence, keeping up with one's skincare regimen, dealing with flare-ups during stressful times, and navigating social situations while obvious symptoms are common obstacles. The development of efficient coping mechanisms and the pursuit of suitable help depend on one's understanding of these issues.

My Path Through Treatment:

A course of trial and error may be required to discover successful therapies for seborrhoeic dermatitis. People typically experiment with various methods to alleviate symptoms and avoid flare-ups, including over-the-counter medicines, prescription drugs, lifestyle adjustments, and alternative therapies. Antifungal creams, corticosteroids, and medicated shampoos are just a few examples of the pharmaceutical and holistic remedies that have been effective for various people; others include changes to one's diet, methods for managing stress, and skincare regimens. Emphasizing the need for individualized treatment programs, it is critical to note that results may vary from patient to patient.

Communities of Support and Advocacy:

Supportive networks and advocacy organizations help ease the burden of living with seborrhoeic dermatitis. These groups allow people to connect, learn about therapies and coping mechanisms, receive emotional support, and work towards a better understanding of the condition. They help people find others who can relate to their struggles and bring them together in a spirit of camaraderie. It is possible to urge recently diagnosed people to seek out these helpful resources by emphasizing the role of advocacy groups and support networks.

Some Words of Wisdom for Patients Who Have Just Received a Diagnosis:

Sharing experiences and insights with others who have dealt with seborrhoeic dermatitis can be a great source of comfort and knowledge for people who have just received a diagnosis. Here are some important things to keep in mind when dealing with seborrhoeic dermatitis: learn about the condition, consult your healthcare provider for a personalized treatment plan, keep up a regular skincare routine, keep stress levels down, reach out to friends and advocacy groups for support, and stay updated on treatment options. Supporting newly diagnosed patients to take it easy and take charge of their health might give them the strength to face their journey head-on.

Reflections on Past Mistakes:

Dealing with seborrhoeic dermatitis daily can teach you a lot about life and what you need to know. Among these lessons could be the significance of being consistent with treatment and self-care, the identification of factors that cause flare-ups, the need to manage symptoms while still enjoying life, the value of standing up for one's healthcare rights, the value of building resilience, and the value of accepting oneself as one's condition. A sense of belonging and mutual support can flourish when people share their experiences to help those going through tough times.

On the Subject of Mental Health:

Seborrhoeic dermatitis affects more than just the skin; it can have a significant psychological and emotional toll as well. As we reflect on our emotional health, we may talk about how we deal with the frustration, shame, or self-consciousness that comes with our visible symptoms; how we handle the stress and anxiety that comes with flare-ups; how we seek professional help when we need it; and how we find ways to be more emotionally resilient and positive overall. Holistic health promotion and addressing the interdependence of mind and body requires acknowledging the emotional components of living with seborrhocic dermatitis.

How it Will Affect Your Personal and Professional Interactions:

Relationships and social interactions can be impacted by seborrhoeic dermatitis in multiple ways. While focusing on self-care, individuals may learn to handle discussions about their illness with loved ones and coworkers, control their reactions to outward symptoms, and keep in touch with friends and family. Realizing the significance of honest communication, establishing limits when necessary, informing others about the disease, and cultivating supportive relationships that encourage understanding and empathy are all part of comprehending the effect on relationships.

Future Aspirations:

Even though seborrhoeic dermatitis makes life difficult, many people still have dreams and ambitions for what the future holds. Our goals include that treatment options will continue to improve, that society will become more aware and understanding of the condition, that healthcare services and support networks will become more accessible, and that we will feel empowered and resilient in managing symptoms and improving our overall well-being. Within the seborrhoeic dermatitis group, sharing aspirations for the future can motivate others and add to a shared vision of improvement and optimism.

Motivational Thoughts:

Themes of perseverance, self-love, empowerment, and unity are frequently highlighted in inspirational messages about seborrhoeic dermatitis. These words have the potential to inspire people to accept and even embrace their path, to reach out for help and knowledge, to stand up for what they need, to revel in even the smallest successes, and to have an optimistic outlook no matter how tough things become

CHAPTER 9

INNOVATING AND USING TECHNOLOGY: A CRITICAL ROLE

Electronic Health Records and Online Consultations:

By facilitating distant discussions between patients and medical professionals, telemedicine has transformed healthcare, particularly dermatology. People suffering from seborrhoeic dermatitis can now get professional guidance and treatment without having to physically visit a clinic. Those in more rural locations, in particular, benefit from virtual consultations because of the increased accessibility, decreased waiting times, and overall convenience they provide.

Portable Self-Monitoring Apps:

The symptoms of seborrhoeic dermatitis can be better managed with the help of mobile apps that record flare-ups, medication compliance, and skincare practices. Better outcomes and more effective communication between patients and healthcare providers are the results of their enabling patients to take an active role in managing their disease.

Dermatology and Wearable Technology:

Seborrhoeic dermatitis-related physiological factors, including skin moisture levels and temperature variations, can be tracked via wearable devices like skin sensors. Early diagnosis of exacerbations and personalized treatment strategies are both made possible with this data.

The Role of AI and ML in the Diagnosis Process:

To aid in the diagnosis of seborrhoeic dermatitis, machine learning algorithms and artificial intelligence (AI) sift through massive databases of dermatological pictures and patient data. Improved diagnostic accuracy, faster evaluations, and decision-making support are all benefits of these technological advancements for the healthcare industry.

Findings from Big Data:

The epidemiology, treatment results, and patient profiles of seborrhoeic dermatitis can be better understood with the use of big data analytics, which extract useful information from massive datasets. Continuous improvement in care delivery is driven by these insights, which inform evidence-based approaches.

Exploring New Drugs and Conducting Clinical Trials:

New drug formulations and tailored therapy are changing the game when it comes to treating seborrhoeic dermatitis. Novel therapeutic approaches are made possible by the evaluation of the safety and effectiveness of novel drugs in clinical trials.

Potential Uses of Nanotechnology:

Targeted medication delivery systems and skin barrier strengthening are two potential dermatological uses of nanotechnology. To maximize therapy efficacy and minimize negative effects, nano-sized particles can penetrate epidermal layers effectively.

Methods for Customised Medical Care:

Genetic factors, microbiome composition, and lifestyle habits are just a few of the particular patient features that personalized medicine takes into account when developing treatment strategies. This method reduces side effects while increasing treatment efficacy.

Important Moral Factors:

Patient confidentiality, data protection, fair technology access, and informed permission for innovative treatments are all important ethical factors to consider when managing seborrhoeic dermatitis. To protect patients' rights and well-being, healthcare practitioners must negotiate these complex ethical landscapes.

Looking Ahead: Potential Paths

With continuous improvements in technology, research, and patient-centered approaches, the future of seborrhoeic dermatitis therapy is bright. Integrated digital platforms for complete dermatological care, precision medicines, and AI-driven predictive models are all possible future advances. To make these potentials a reality and improve outcomes for people with seborrhoeic dermatitis, stakeholders must continue to collaborate.

CHAPTER 10

VIEWS FROM AROUND THE WORLD ON SEBORRHOEIC DERMATITIS

Global Incidence Rates

People of all ages can be affected with seborrhoeic dermatitis, a skin ailment that is common worldwide. Depending on where you look and who you ask, the prevalence percentages can be anywhere from 1% to 5% in adults and much more in babies. Healthcare systems can better distribute resources and adapt treatment plans to meet the unique demands of each region when they have a good grasp of these prevalence rates.

Disparities in Health Care Delivery by Region

Factors like healthcare accessibility, cultural customs, and environmental impacts might cause regional variations in the diagnosis and management of seborrhoeic dermatitis. While some areas may have defined treatment protocols and diagnostic criteria, others may struggle to get a proper diagnosis and may not have easy access to specialists. Improving patient outcomes and guaranteeing equitable healthcare delivery requires addressing these differences.

Traditional Values and Customs

How people from different cultural backgrounds view and treat seborrhoeic dermatitis might vary greatly. For instance, there may be a lag in diagnosis and treatment because some cultures value traditional cures more than medical methods. To build trust within various populations and offer culturally competent care, healthcare providers must understand and respect these cultural subtleties.

The Influence of Socioeconomic Factors

The management, diagnosis, and prevalence of seborrhoeic dermatitis are all significantly impacted by socioeconomic circumstances. Inadequate health education, financial limitations, and limited access to health care can all lead to unequal disease outcomes. Improving healthcare access and providing reasonable treatment choices are key efforts to remove socioeconomic obstacles and reduce the incidence of seborrhoeic dermatitis worldwide.

Disparities in Healthcare Accessibility

Geographical obstacles, inadequate healthcare infrastructure, and labor shortages are all examples of healthcare accessibility challenges that might delay the diagnosis and treatment of seborrhoeic dermatitis. Improving access to dermatological treatment, particularly in neglected regions, requires concerted action by healthcare providers, governmental agencies, and nonprofit groups.

Partnerships in Dermatology on a Global Scale

Dermatology research, practice exchange, and patient care results related to seborrhoeic dermatitis and other skin disorders might greatly benefit from international collaborations. Knowledge sharing, healthcare provider training, and the creation of evidence-based guidelines specific to varied populations are all made possible through collaborative projects.

Policy Shifts and Advocacy

Raising awareness, obtaining research funding, and encouraging equitable access to dermatological treatment are all greatly aided by advocacy activities and changes in legislation. It is crucial to involve stakeholders, advocacy groups, and lawmakers to establish policies that promote seborrhoeic dermatitis early diagnosis, appropriate treatment, and patient education programs.

Initiatives for Funding Research

To drive innovation, advance scientific understanding, and discover new therapeutics for seborrhoeic dermatitis, research funding projects are crucial. Improvements in patient outcomes and quality of life can be achieved by increased funding in dermatology research, which can lead to breakthroughs in disease causes, biomarker identification, and personalized therapy methods.

Healthcare Professionals' Educational Programmes

Improving diagnostic accuracy, treatment efficacy, and patient-centered care for seborrhoeic dermatitis requires educational programs for healthcare professionals, such as dermatologists, primary care doctors, and nurses. The most up-to-date evidence-based practices and recommendations can be accessed by healthcare practitioners through continuing medical education programs, seminars, and internet sites.

A World Free of Dermatitis: Our Vision

A world free of dermatitis requires concerted efforts to eliminate seborrhoeic dermatitis and other skin disorders through improved diagnosis, treatment, and prevention. Promoting public awareness, interdisciplinary collaborations, research funding, and policies that prioritize skin health as a global public health priority are all part of this vision. Our shared goal is to create an environment where people from all walks of life can obtain the best dermatological care possible so they can have beautiful, healthy skin.